Highly Intuitive People

The Ultimate Guide For Mastering Your Gift (Highly Sensitive, Empath, Life Changing, Survival Manual, Relationships)

Kristine S. Everest

Table of Contents

1 - Introduction

Instinct

You live in a world that fuels your instinct. Numbers, theories, frameworks, and logic have very little place in your mind. That is the life of the highly intuitive.

Your past and upbringing have allowed you to nourish the other side of human capacity. You live on the other side of intellect. It's not the losing side, it's just the other side. It's the side that has kept us alive during the stone ages. It's the side that has allowed us to outlive the dinosaurs.

But what good is that side today; in a world that prizes intellect and gives laurels to the learned? What place is there for those that learn from their instinct? For those who trust their guts and their hearts more than their mind?

This is what this book is for. This book is here to tell you that your gift is not a curse. It is a rare blessing that will help you grow in an untold number of ways. You just need to awaken it and hone it to serve you.

This book will walk you through understanding and controlling your gift. It doesn't matter how long you've been living with your talents. Here, you will come to love what you have as it will help you get through life.

You may be in the dark about your talents or you may already be at peace with what makes you special; it doesn't matter. This book is designed to make you appreciate what you have and help you get the most out of your work, family, and other personal relationships. You won't just become more intuitive. You'll become an emotional beacon and stronghold for other people that do not share your talents.

2 - Understanding the Gift

It was the late Steve Jobs that tried to define the side of intuition. According to the founder of one of the biggest tech brands in the world, intuitiveness is a more natural form of human adaptability.

The iconic Carl Jung was one of those who attempted to label this capacity. According to him, people are divided into two sets. There are those who operate with logic and reason, questioning the environment, and using their knowledge to guide their decisions.

On the other hand, there are people like you; people with the gift. These are people with internal responses that come from instinct. Some experts would call it "thinking without thinking."

It's another facet of human intelligence that usually gets ignored in some of the more developed parts of the world. But in other areas such as India and other rural sections, intuitiveness has a greater importance than intellect. But what is intuitiveness? How is it different from other forms of intelligence?

Intuition Defined

The dictionary defines intuition as the capacity to understand a concept immediately, sans the logical reasoning.

In simpler terms, it's knowing something based on that gut feeling. You don't see any signs of danger, yet you know something bad is about to happen. You've barely known a person for five minutes but you know they're a good person. You've been in a room with someone for barely a minute and you already know something is bothering them.

These are examples of intuition. Don't be mistaken to think that it's an exclusive gift that only a select few people enjoy. It's a capacity everyone has. It's just that it's heightened and more developed in some more than others. Are you one of those people?

Intuition is not blind guesswork. It's something more than just claiming something and hoping it to be correct. It has a deeper and more profound connection with your senses and your feelings.

The funny part about intuition is that you yourself can't explain why you know these things. Has that ever happened to you? Just saying "I just feel it" when trying to explain your opinions to someone? That's just one of the many things that set intuitive people apart from the rest.

Telling If You Are Intuitive

What else sets you apart? What are those subtle differences you've noticed in you as you grew up and interacted with other people? According to experts, the highly intuitive do things differently and show signs of their gut prowess.

They Root Themselves in the Moment

The mind of the intuitive absorbs everything with their senses. The environment feeds their guts. They take note of what they see, hear, smell, and feel. Every little detail comes into their minds and creates a mental image that only they can see.

These sensations come together in their minds and help them act on rational impulses. Do you look around and take note of things? Are you tallying the general count of the people in the area? Do you immediately become aware of places with a lot of people? Can you immediately tell from which direction certain sounds are coming from?

As an intuitive individual, your gift requires you to gather information about your surroundings as soon as you put both feet on the ground. Your tendency to look around and observe comes as second nature. You're someone who "smells" danger even from a distance. You're also the last person to relax upon arrival at a new and unfamiliar place.

They Talk to Themselves

Highly intuitive people are not crazy; they just have an "inner voice" with which they have conversations. Some people call it a conscience. Others call it their guardian angel. Whatever name you have for it, you have a second-self inside of you, helping you process what you're feeling.

And no, the highly intuitive don't talk to themselves loudly while they converse with their impulses. They have silent discussions about their environments. They discern and determine what they're feeling at that certain moment.

Have you had many discussions with your inner voice? How many arguments have you had with yourself about how you feel and what you should do? You're no loner, but you value the time of self-reflection to enrich your impulsive nature.

In fact, you probably set aside a certain time of the day just to be alone with your thoughts. It could be while you prepare your breakfast. It could also be while you're in the shower. It may even be during your commute or drive to work and back home.

Those times are important to you. This is where you have those important discussions with yourself. That is your natural environment.

They Are Profound Thinkers

In line with talking to themselves, the highly intuitive can reach deep levels of thought because they always have someone on which to bounce their ideas. Your personal conversations with yourself don't just always end with close-ended thoughts.

You get deep into the why of the things you're feeling. At your very core, you don't just want to accept what you're feeling. You want to understand why you're feeling a certain way as well.

Do you always reroute your thoughts from your decisions all the way to a central principle you hold dear to yourself? Have you always gone back to your core values every time you need to make a choice? Do you always double back from opportunities just to make sure your feelings and principles aren't compromised?

Because of this trait, intuitive people are the best people to approach when it comes to life decisions. This is because these people are beyond just weighing the pros and cons. For you, personal happiness, satisfaction, and even fulfillment become important factors to consider, further complicating discussions. This allows you to really get into someone's skin and find out what really makes someone happy.

They are Attuned with their Subconscious

Although the subconscious mind is beyond the grasp and understanding of many, the intuitive person cherishes the links they have between their waking minds and their automated consciousness.

Have you ever woken up from a dream and knew that it was your body trying to tell you something about yourself? As a highly intuitive individual, you understand that you have feelings and urges buried underneath your waking thoughts which only come to life when you sleep.

And when you're intuitive, you don't just have foggy visions when you dream. When you dream, you dream vividly. Details come with crystal clarity, allowing you to recall almost any detail the moment you wake up.

When this happens, you start to dig deep. Being the profound thinker that you are, you try to find meaning in these experiences and learn a little more about yourself with every dream you have.

They Never Bottle Their Feelings

For the intuitive, feelings aren't just excuses to cry or to act a certain way. Feelings are messages from our subconscious, trying to tell us what we deeply desire.

Those who are restrained by what other people think will try their best to hide their real feelings at the risk of being judged. You, on the other hand, openly embrace what you feel and enjoy a true openness with yourself.

Have you ever been stifled by a situation wherein you're expected to feel a certain way but you feel the opposite? You don't go with the stifling. You go against it and accept what you're feeling at that moment, recognizing it to be what's true.

They are Eternal Optimists

Since intuitive people are well-versed with what they feel and how to process these feelings, they're also better-equipped at dealing with setbacks and negative emotions.

You must have felt the same way at certain points in your life. You're not one to give in to wallowing but you're capable of accepting setbacks and loss. At the same time, you're also a firm believer of moving and welcoming new experiences to replace bad ones.

They Understand Purpose

Due to their love for profound thoughts, intuitive people appreciate the bigger picture in life. They know that their experiences lead to personal discoveries about themselves and that leads them towards a specific direction.

That is probably the reason you're reading this manual. Are you trying to find a purpose with your gift? What was it meant to do in your life? Where will this talent lead you? Better yet, where will you take your gifts once you know how to harness them?

They Are Sensitive to Others

Finally, their talents allow them to gain inklings if not glimpses of how other people around them are feeling. The highly intuitive are ideal empaths that can sense the general aura of an area and the people within.

Have you ever felt a change in mood without warning? Has the cold breath of negativity suddenly come over you despite your good temperament at that moment? You've probably picked up someone else's emotions.

Your observation of the environment and people lead you to ideas about how other people are behaving. Again, it's not guesswork. You feel it. You can sense their joy, hesitation, anger, and even sadness when you're with someone.

If you've come around these signs in your life, there's a big chance that you're highly intuitive. You pick up the subtleties that most people overlook in exchange for a different perspective.

3 - Types of Intuition

Just as there are different types of intellects, there are also different forms of intuition. They all manifest the same kind of knowledge, it's just that the method of delivery is different. Your gift may be prone to one kind more than another, but that doesn't mean it isn't useful.

Audio-Based Intuition

People who possess this type of intuition have deep and meaningful discussions within themselves. They've mastered this art so well that the voice inside their heads is very audible.

They use this voice as a guide which gives them their hunches in the form of straight messages.

- No

- Don't

- Go

- Yes

- Think

- Check

These are some examples of what they hear when their intuition kicks in. Their bodies and minds are wired to communicate with them using these short messages. These people claim they can really hear someone else speak to them, giving them advice on how to proceed.

Image-Based Intuition

If you have people who hear their hunches, there are also those who manifest their instinct in the form of images.

For this type, they can either dream of scenarios of suddenly conjure up a mental image of what they think might happen or what course of action they should take. It's a personal image for them that may or may not be symbolic in nature.

Sometimes, they still need to figure out the meaning of their images. Other times, they get specific answers. It all depends on how well they've honed their skills and how attuned they are with their bodies.

Sensation-Based Intuition

This is probably the most common form of intuition but certainly not the least useful. Here, intuitive people get their hunches from certain sensations that they experience. This is a broad approach which could have many possible out-lets.

Their hunches could come in the form of butterflies in the stomach. It could also be a sudden wave of depression that comes over them for no reason at all. It may even be a sudden shot of pain through their temples.

These types of people use these sensations in relation to their situation. Immediately, they attribute what they're feeling to what is happening around them. Hence, they can zero in on their hunches.

Cognitive-Based Intuition

Finally, there are the types where their hunches set into their minds with ease. These kinds of intuitive people gain complete and specific thoughts. When they encounter someone, they can tell if these people are going through something or if they're about to do something drastic.

At the same time, their gift also gives them insight into what other people are feeling at that moment. Their hunches are a little more specific than other types, but this is the rarest of them all.

Usually, experts and psychics that have finely honed their skills are able to practice this form of intuition. Years and years of development and research will lead you to training your intuition to immediately give you full thoughts instead of feelings and images.

The Life of the Gifted

Yes, you have gifts that set you apart from others, but everything comes at a price. Being highly intuitive is not easy. Despite being special, you have myriad adjustments to make to yourself to adapt to the demands of the present day. That may not always be a walk in the park for you.

The Struggles of The Intuitive

Since you see the world differently, the way you interact with people is also different. One of the most difficult things you will experience as an intuitive person is explaining yourself to other people.

How do you convince someone that you're right when all you're working on are your feelings and intuition?

In a world where logic is prized, you may find it hard to get your points and ideas across. This could cause misunderstandings with most people. This creates a need for you to widen your understanding and strengthen your patience with people who aren't ready to understand you on your level.

In turn, this skill becomes even harder to practice with people that want to take advantage of you. Given your natural talents, you can easily tell if people are telling you lies to win you over.

When this happens, it's difficult to remain civil and reciprocate their fake niceness. You know better than anyone the importance of honesty as you value it with yourself. How do you treat someone who isn't being honest with you at face value?

If you were to call someone out, what proof do you have? Intuitions are weak in terms of logic. How do you tell someone that they aren't being honest without offending them? How do you inform someone of their self-destructive behavior without ruining your relationship with them?

Because of these nuances, you may find it easier to keep your feelings and thoughts to yourself. This may cause you to shut yourself off from most people. In some cases, you could even be shutting out the people that care about you out of fear of misunderstanding.

This habit causes us to look inward most of the time with a pessimistic eye. We then become overly-sensitive of what we're thinking; to the point that we think it's wrong. In our quest for understanding, we end up misunderstanding our own talents and take our insights for granted.

Most intuitive people cling to a life of introversion. For them, meeting new people is an experience that requires energy.

Being social creatures, we still need human interaction. But for the introverted intuitive, it's more than just a meeting. For them, it's already a call to see if they can bond with someone on an emotional and intellectual level. That's why it costs them energy.

Unlike extroverts, introverts draw their energy from their past experiences and their alone time. This is one of the reasons why it's important for talented individuals like yourself to partake in some form of meditation.

Introverts use this energy when they interact with other people. This is because they dig deep and share their thoughts with others. It's not because they've become attached, but because that's how they get to know someone else.

For them, small talk is a rudimentary waste of time. Some of the greatest intuitive people are self-confessed introverts. Look at J.K. Rowling, author of the iconic figure of Harry Potter and his myriad wizarding world that has charmed millions.

For her, small talk is boring and she considers herself inadequate for such things. She couldn't even speak to a stranger to borrow a pen.

You may have had similar experiences as well. Have you ever considered just keeping to yourself despite having a need that could be answered by reaching out to a stranger? Do social gatherings tire you out? Does the solace and privacy of your own space outshine even the largest of parties? It's probably because you're intuitive.

In addition to that, we get lost in our own frustrations and end up belittling the things that we can do for ourselves and others. It's this large mix-up of feelings that could lead you down the wrong path of development. Hence, it's important to understand your gift and what makes it stand above the rest.

4 - The Advantages of The Highly Intuitive

Of course, if there are reasons to fear your gifts, there are also reasons to celebrate. Your talents aren't just for display. These are real-life advantages that give you benefits you cannot get anywhere else.

First off, you're better protected against those with malicious intent. This is because you can smell that from a mile away. You can see it in the way someone talks to you; and how they act towards your responses. You don't have to test them. You know they have ulterior motives.

This tells of untold advantages, to begin with. With your gift, you become an ideal judge of character. In business, that has untold benefits. You know who to trust and who to ignore. In relationships, you know where to invest your time and emotions. With friends, you get to filter who you should keep in your life.

Next, to that comes emotional intelligence. Take note, you're not emotional. You're emotionally intelligent. Those are two different things. One is a poorly-induced state of mind while the other is a hard-earned mental discipline.

This means you're aware of the presence of negativity in your life but at the same time, you're capable of letting these things influence you only up to a certain point.

With that, you move on faster. You get your life back earlier than most people. Don't misunderstand, though. As an intuitive person, you're not immune to the struggles of daily life. It's just that you're better equipped to handle these things compared to other people.

In addition to that, your capacity to deal with multitudes of emotions makes you an ideally-creative spirit. With all these feelings and ideas locked up inside, most intuitive people seek refuge in the release offered by the creative arts.

You could be entangled in music, the written word, film, acting and even painting! It doesn't matter what kind of art form you pursue. If it provides you with the creative expression you desire, you will embrace it with all your heart.

Another facet that your gifts give you is a firm resolution. The highly intuitive simply abhor standing on figurative sand.

As a person that takes everything into account, you can't stand not thinking things through. You may be prone to overthinking but you're not one to be caught doing something you haven't thought about. For you, every decision is a firm one. When you commit to something, you give it your all because you've thought about it for countless times.

This makes you a great role model for others who can't seem to find their footing. Your commitment to your decisions is unlike any other, and this is all because you know how important it is to fully believe in something.

But what sets apart your gifts the most is your natural sensitivity to special life events. Because of your heightened emotions and control, you feel things on a deeper level than most people. The joy you feel is higher, as is your pleasure.

For you, a home-cooked meal isn't just a gastronomic trip. It's an act of love that fills your soul just as much as your belly. Experiences are very potent and important things for you.

And it's not just with food and get-togethers. Highly-intuitive people also enjoy more pleasure when it comes to sex. This is because making love doesn't just trigger physical cues for attachment. It also sets off emotional signals to create deep and lasting relationships.

5 - Survival Tips for the Gifted

On top of appreciating life and all its splendor, a big challenge poses itself on you every day. How will you make the right decisions with the right people and grow as an individual?

In a world where logic is valued in business and even in relationships, intuitive people may find it difficult to adjust to their environments and the people around them.

It's important for people like you to pick up on some tips to help improve the quality of your life.

Weed Out the Toxic People

First, determine who has what power over how you feel. Yes, the way you feel is something under your control, but there are people whose constant negativity and incurable misery will immediately seep into your good mood and turn things around.

These are known as toxic people. They infect you by giving off negative signals, feeding your intuition and poisoning your demeanor. You've probably met a few of these people already.

It could be that friend who always asks for advice for a miserable problem but does the exact opposite of what you say. It could be that in-law who is never happy with anything that you do. It could also be your romantic partner who has grown cold towards you.

Given your natural sensitivity, it's hard to ignore the influence of these people. If you work with them or live with them, their influence just grows in intensity. Take note of these people in your life.

When you've identified them, start avoiding them if you can't help them. Of course, the first thing you would want to do is to assist in improving their disposition in life, but if they've been miserable long enough, there's little even a gifted individual such as yourself can accomplish with them.

You don't need that kind of negativity in your life; especially in a life like yours. You could be enjoying such a lovely day with the best possible news you could ever receive but have it all taken away with one encounter with the wrong person. Your gifts could do that to you. Those people could do that to you.

You also want to save your energy and effort for the people

that matter. When you've labeled all the toxic people in your life, it leaves out the important people. These are the people who have proven themselves to be a positive influence in your life. And even if these people affect your negatively from time to time, they're the ones that deserve your attention.

Create a Habit of Thought-Watching

With your active imagination of complex thought processes, it's necessary for you to develop a habit of checking your train of thought. You may not like where your thoughts take you from time to time.

You could be in the middle of a stream of disappointment for a day which could then lead to chronic depression if you're not careful with the things that cross your mind.

On that same note, you could also be so happy that you're blinded from other issues that require your attention. You could get sometimes carried away by your thoughts that you miss the bigger picture, and intuitive individuals are all about the bigger picture.

When you notice yourself brooding over something, take a step back and examine your thoughts. Ask yourself some probing questions to prove to yourself that what you're doing is not in your best interest.

- What am I thinking?

- Where will these thoughts take me?

- Am I brooding over this too much?

- Am I being melodramatic here?

- How will these thoughts help me get better?

Answering these questions will help you shift your focus towards a more positive goal and stop you from falling into emotional pits from which there is little escape.

On the same topic, it's also important to make an affirmation that you're changing your thoughts for the better. Claiming something within your mind can be a very powerful tool. Simply saying "This is not right. I will get better" to yourself is almost as good as doing it in real life; especially for someone like you. This is because mental messages to yourself are more powerful even than spoken words.

Practice Forgiveness

Just as the old saying goes, to err is human. To forgive, divine.

For the genuine intuitive person, slights and grudges are commonplace in our minds. You're the type who will never forget a good time had with friends. By that same virtue, you will also never forget a wrong that has been done to you.

It also gets deeper the more it hurts you. When you let your emotions get the best of you, you can't help but think about things more and more. You fill yourself with negative thoughts in an effort to console yourself when you're convinced that you're the victim.

When this happens, your behavior changes. You become mistrustful and distant, even from those that want to help you. This is because you've created a wall of hate that you've built so well with your developed emotions.

Naturally, you're the only one who can take down this wall; and it is done through forgiveness. And that is easier said than done.

A big weakness of intuitive people is that they have a hard time letting go of things that mean a lot to them. Whether it's bad or good, if it struck a nerve of strum a heartstring, you hold on to these things with such vigor.

And as you hold on to your anger and your desire to get even, you forget that you're also doing wrong to yourself. You're not letting yourself grow in your talents.

When you forgive, you don't just give other people the chance to move on. You give yourself the amazing opportunity to learn from your experiences and be an example to other people.

You get stuck on ideas of hatred because you no longer see the benefits of forgiving people. The central idea in your head in anger is getting even. You want to see justice meted out. You want to see karma in action. You believe that when it happens, you will be satisfied.

This couldn't be further from the truth. Even if karma came around the corner and tit-for-tat is complete, you're still just going to be as miserable as ever. It get even worse over time because the longer to persist on an idea, the more likely it is to become a truth with you.

Have a "Safe Space"

If meditation and clearing your thoughts are important to the mind, then you should have a designated place for meditation at home.

It doesn't have to be a full room with electronics and speakers and diffusers. It's an ideal place, but not necessary. All you need is a small corner wherein you can affirm no negative thoughts will enter.

Some people will call it their happy place. Some call it their quiet corner. It doesn't matter what name you call it. What matters is that nothing negative should enter that space, because that is where you hone your thoughts and realign your focus.

When you step into that space, you should be prepared for meditation and relaxation.

It can be next to your bed or a corner of your bed. It could also be a small corner of your room. It can also be right underneath your shower head. This place should hold a very special place in your heart and it doesn't have to make sense to other people. In fact, you shouldn't let other people with negative thoughts into that space if they aren't meditating with you.

Maintain a Feeling of Gratitude

This works wonders even for those who aren't "gifted". Many successful people from likes of Einstein, Warren Buffet, Charlie Munger, J.K. Rowling and even Steve Jobs emphasize how important it is to be thankful.

And it's not just being thankful to your god. It's also being thankful to the people that have helped you get the things that you need and want.

When you're thankful, there's no room for resentment, anger, jealousy, and pride. You are humbled just to the right level. In such a state, much can be achieved.

You work harder. You enjoy working hard to show respect to your benefactors. You eliminate competition from your mind. You're clear of malice and your focus is unshakable under the premise of personal shame.

Which is why it's a good idea to think of things for which you're thankful before starting your day. It sets the mood of the day and empowers you to take on whatever challenges that lie ahead of you.

Love Your Gift Like a Child Loves a Toy

Yes, you're special. Yes, you can do, see, feel, and experience things that many people cannot. Despite that, it doesn't mean that you are part of an elite group of people that segregate themselves from society. In more interesting cases, intuitive people such as yourself are the ones that are segregated negatively because of your unique insights.

Your talents are not for show only. They are meant to enrich your life and the lives of those around you. Your gifts aren't meant to make other people jealous. They are meant to make other people stronger.

With that thought in mind, don't treat your talents like a prized stallion that you spoil daily with ridiculous customs and rules. It won't grow that way.

Instead, love your gift the way a child loves their toys. They play with them lovingly, enjoying every second of entertainment and joy they get. They devote their time and attention to shaping their imaginations with their toys, creating small worlds that only they know about.

On the same note, they will take their toys to the mud, to the dirt and even to the streets if they could. You should do the same with your gifts. They should be with you and used whenever you can.

6 - Honing the Gift

Just like any other talent, your intuition fades into obscurity when it is not practiced. Yes, it will always be there, dormant at times, but it would be a shame not to develop your skills and live life to the fullest.

Interestingly, how do you develop something that doesn't follow a rational or logical process? Traditional methods may not be suitable for such a gift. What you need are modern-day approaches.

Mindfulness Meditation

As simple as this sounds, this may well be one of the most difficult forms of meditation to master. This is not because of religious or spiritual ties. In fact, mindfulness has nothing to do with these concepts.

At its very core, mindfulness is the capacity to channel your focus on the moment. This is something almost anyone can achieve with the proper guidance. You don't need to follow a specific philosophy or preach a certain faith. All you need to do is to live in your present state.

That may be easier said than done. Whether we admit it or not, we are all residents of our own thoughts. These thoughts could sometimes hinder us from living in the moment.

This is especially true today. We live in a world full of issues and challenges that cloud our minds and keep us locked in our desires. I want this. I want that. When will it happen? It's easy to become lost in a self-destructive dialogue with yourself.

Interestingly, quieting this inner dialogue will help sharpen your intuition. Yes, it was mentioned that the intuitive are great with their inner dialogue. Despite that, your inner voice could lead you astray as you try to figure out things.

Mindfulness meditation will help you realign your sights and clean your mental slate. Fortunately, it doesn't take years to master. In fact, you can do it right now.

Before putting down this book to practice, read these instructions carefully. Find a place in which to meditate. It doesn't have to be a spiritual area in which meditation is usually done. This doesn't even have to be at a church or a temple.

Finding a quiet corner of the room with a comfortable chair will suffice. When looking for a spot, it's important that there should be as little audible and visual distractions as possible. Meditating in a busy and hectic area can be difficult.

Once you've found a place in which to meditate, place yourself in a comfortable position. The good thing about this is that you can choose to either lean back into a reclining chair or to completely lie down. The choice is up to your preferences.

In a comfortable position, you can now begin a short mindfulness meditation sequence. This shouldn't take more than five minutes to complete.

Begin the sequence by closing your eyes. Mindfulness meditation is a process wherein you empty your thoughts and absorb your environment. This means the first thing you should do is to recognize the thoughts you're harboring at that moment and let it go.

As soon as you close your eyes, try to paint yourself a mental image of your breath. This task alone should help you clear your thoughts. Try to imagine your lungs expand and decompress with each breath you take.

Remember to keep your eyes closed as you breathe. To

make things more vivid, picture your breath as it enters your body, finding its way into your lungs and mixing with your blood. Feel yourself become refreshed with every breath.

At the same time, also take note that your head feels lighter with every breath you take. Don't worry if your body moves around a lot as you breathe in and breathe out. That's part of the experience.

Don't even worry about the method of breathing that you're using. As long as it's comfortable, keep whatever pace you want. What's important is that you're paying attention to only your breathing.

After a few breaths, you will notice that you cannot stop yourself from not breathing. This is a sign that tells you your body has shifted breathing from a subconscious activity to a conscious one. You now should tell yourself to breathe. Don't be alarmed by this. It's a sign that means your meditation is going as planned.

As you begin to relax, you will also find that your thoughts may start drifting. You may start going back to whatever it is you were thinking before meditating. This is also a natural error that a lot of beginners make.

When this happens, take another deep breath and realign your focus towards your breathing. The purpose of this activity is to help you clear your mind, not help you think about something else.

As you feel your head getting lighter from the breathing, ease into your position and continue visualizing your breath as it nourishes you. As you get more relaxed, you're telling your body to stop implementing its stress responses and that you're safe.

You'll now you're done meditating when you've realized that you're no longer stressed and have a more positive demeanor at the end of the activity. At this point, don't just open your eyes and abruptly end the meditation, that's one way to waste all that time you've spent meditating.

Instead, take one last breath and slowly open your eyes as you exhale. You will notice that your perspective of your environment has changed a bit and things seem a little brighter. That is how mindfulness works.

Other Forms

You'll be pleased to know that this short activity is just one of many mindfulness exercises that you can do on your own. The one you just finished is known as mindfulness breathing.

Other ways you can practice mindfulness also include body inspections. Instead of focusing on your breathing, you turn your focus towards what the various parts of your body are feeling.

This is done by making mental notes of the sensations that your skin encounters. What are your hands feeling? How does the fabric of your clothes feel against your skin? What sensations are your feet feeling while they're inside your shoes? Answering these questions as you meditate can help shift your focus and clear your mind.

These are known as body checks. More advanced users put together combinations of body checks and breathing meditations to get the most out of their quiet time. The longer you practice your mindfulness, the easier it will become for you to achieve harmony with your inner voice.

7 - Journal Maintenance

You may be hesitant about the apparent worth of a journal to an intuitive person, but nothing could be more enriching than a written collection of your personal thoughts.

Most people consider the act of keeping a journal a tiresome one. For the talented intuitive person, a journal is a logbook of the soul. With a journal, you get to give you inner voice a physical form.

This method of honing your talents doesn't follow the same route as conventional journal-writing. For the intuitive, journal keeping is a chance to let your mind free and wreak havoc on a clean sheet of paper.

Primarily, you don't really need a fancy journal or a diary to begin. You just need a notebook on which you can write. From there, the magic begins.

Before diving in, be sure to mark the date and time of your writing. It really helps you piece your thoughts together when you are more specific with your time.

As you begin your entry, try not to pay too much attention to a central theme and motif. The purpose of a journal is to let your thoughts run wild, not to create a preconceived idea. That will only frustrate you as you write.

When starting, don't worry about the first few words that come out. They're usually what gets the ball rolling. You can start with almost anything. Try asking yourself a question and see where your inner dialogue takes you.

Don't get frustrated if your work isn't something appealing to the immediate reader. Your writing there isn't meant for the eyes of other people. It's more of a tool you can use to reflect patterns in your thinking. It helps you see if you've been circling around a repeating concept or idea. It will also tell you if you're going through chronic stress over time.

Another interesting facet of journal-keeping is that you can also use it as a dream-log. Other people call it a dream-journal but the concept remains the same. Besides setting aside a good hour every day to scribble your inner conversations, you can also use a journal to capture your dreams before you forget them throughout the day.

8 - Indulging The Other Senses

Many experts refer to your intuition as the "sixth sense" which encompasses knowledge gained from all our 5 sense organs. Interestingly, developing these rudimentary senses is a great way to develop your intuition.

You may not notice it fully, but feedback from your senses fuels your instinct. This works similarly to the way animals detect danger in their environment. Take note that they don't just use their eyes to gauge threats. Some animals are even sensitive to precipitation in the air to watch out for storms.

This then leads to a unique question. How do you pay attention and sharpen your senses?

Using principles from mindfulness meditation, honing your senses requires you to ground yourself in a moment to assess the sensations around you. Placing yourself in experiences with diverse sensory stimuli will help promote such growth.

Pay attention to your senses as you experience things. Sitting back on a massage chair is certainly a comfortable experience. In that chair, try to determine which body parts of yours are getting attention from the chair. What sort of alleviation are you feeling? Is it releasing tension? Is it relaxing your muscles?

Do the same thing with a good meal. Does it just taste good? Try to segregate the flavors you're experiencing. Are you detecting hints of your favorite ingredients? What elements of your meal do you find most striking in your dish? How well do the dishes complement each other on your palette?

On the same note, sharpen your sense of smell by exposing yourself to various aromas. Aromatherapy is an ideal way to de-stress and sample the fragrant scents of various flowers and plants. Acquainting yourself with these scents will broaden your sensory vocabulary and leave you refreshed at the same time.

Take this process to every sensory experience you have. The best thing about this is that you're always going through sensations. It's just a matter of finding the right moments to practice.

One of the best ways to bombard your senses is to go hiking. You don't necessarily have to climb a mountain to experience something good. Sometimes, a good walk at the park will suffice. Being one with nature allows you to hone these senses, just as Mother Nature intended for us.

Note Your Body Signals

Different people have different descriptions of a "gut feeling". For some, their innards twist up and they get restless when something is about to go wrong. For others, butterflies in their stomach start to form in anticipation for something.

How does your body communicate with you? What sort of signals does it give? This is where keeping a journal comes in very handy. As you age and mature, your body develops different kinds of telling signals to alert you of your intuition. Writing them down will give you a better guide to understanding yourself.

The only way for you to get opportunities to read your body is when you're forced to rely on your intuition. Go on an adventure. Better yet, plan an adventure. Even if you haven't left yet, the experience of putting together a trip makes you feel all sorts of emotions as you make decisions.

As you plan, take note of how your intuition communicates. Do you twist up when you think about certain places? Do you get queasy as you consider visiting some in-laws out of state? Do you feel relaxed as you target going to the hometown of a childhood friend? Take note of these things as you plan and as you travel.

Additionally, the break from routine will help liven up your senses. Nothing is better at dulling a sharp knife than repeated use. Breaking away from the drudgery of everyday life is a good way to immerse yourself in experiences that will sharpen your instinct.

Unleash Your Creativity

One of the biggest reasons why intuitive people are creative is because they appreciate their artistic outlets. Who better to enjoy the creative release of creation that someone that embodies the very notion of creativity?

Being an intuitive person, you are a breeding ground for ideas. Simple concepts turn into complex patterns for you, waiting to be expressed. When something hits you, it comes just as suddenly as one of your hunches. They are unplanned, therefore, meaningful.

Your stories, experiences, and emotions make for great creative material. Even if you're currently bereft of inspiration, your intuition floods you with possibilities. You just need to be open enough to see them as they come to you.

The best part about this is that the more you express yourself, the more attuned you become to your creative tendencies. The better you understand your emotion. You go deeper into yourself, learning more as you reach the apex of your creativity.

Never Force It

There are times when you literally need your intuition to step in and it doesn't come to you. It could as you sit in front of that job offer. It could also be when you're talking to that person who's trying to borrow money from you.

When your instincts don't kick it, it can be frustrating; like never being able to find a pen when you need one. When this happens, you prod yourself, blaming your inadequacy. This is no way to hone your talents.

According to psychics and other experts, intuition is more likely to take place when you're calm and relaxed. Remember that this talent springs from a deep and satisfying relationship between your waking mind and your subconscious.

With that being said, it is necessary to recognize your stress signals and to work on clearing your mind so that your instincts kick in with more efficiency. On top of that, you get clearer messages and hunches in a relaxed state rather than an agitated one.

Appreciate the benefits of approaching every situation with a calm mind. It's a concept that works well for both the logical mind as well as the intuitive one. Reasoning and feeling work better when you're not clouded by thoughts of frustration and confusion.

On the other hand, it's important to also recognize the difference between apathy and calmness. Your gifts don't require you to lose concern in order for them to work. They require you to understand the value and weight of your situation and to look at things through a disciplined perspective. You don't need razor-sharp focus to work your intuition; just a relaxed state of mind.

Testing Your Intuition

What other way is there to practice a skill than to use it in real life situations?

Putting your intuition into practical use may be easier than you think. Take the news, for instance. It is full of people, events, and emotions for you to read. You just have to use a different eye when watching.

Take a certain politician, for example. Let's say that this politician is involved in a big controversy that affects his public standing. Being a public figure, this person needs to make a statement or take a certain course of action.

Tap into your intuition and try to get a feel of what this person might too. It's not plain guesswork if that's what you're thinking. It's more of hypothesis-creation.

Look at this person and try to see what they're feeling. Shame and frustration could be good places to start. Try to dig deeper and see how they work. You also have access to this person's history, with them being a politician.

Take those things into account and say what you would do if you were in their position. Would you come clean? Would you deny? Would you blame someone else? Would you step down from office? Would you just disappear? There are so many options available. And using your gift, your guess will probably be just as close as what will happen in real life.

Even if that isn't the case, you can still learn from your mistakes. Compare what you've thought of to what really happens. From there, you can see what points you might have overlooked. From that point, it's just a matter of adjusting your thought process to make more accurate readings.

If you're not a fan of the news, you can also practice on the people around you. Be with other people, even if you're not talking to them. Observe them as they go about their daily routine. Are you noticing changes in their behavior? Are they exhibiting something out of the ordinary? You may want to talk to them and learn more. You'll be surprised at what you can learn.

It is through these activities that you can better acquaint yourself with your gift. The more you use it, the better and sharper it gets. With enough practice, you'll be able to see things from a mile away.

9 - Intuition Vs Naivete

Whether you're a beginner with your talents or a veteran with your gifts, you will have come across the notion that your intuition could be nothing more than your own vanity.

One of the biggest challenges faced by any intuitive person is to see the value in their own gifts and look beyond what other people say about them. And mind you, people will say a lot of things.

- "You're lucky."

- "You cheated."

- "You're talking to someone on the inside."

When other people doubt your intuition, there's a good chance you'll start doubting it as well. It's easy to ask for logic from something that doesn't need logic to operate in the first place. And when someone asks you to explain how you know these things, you tend to lose credibility when you say "I just know these things."

Trusting Yourself

This is the first thing you need to do. Accept the fact that your gut feeling is trying to tell you something and that it doesn't want to lead you astray. Yes, you're in control of your own body. Your senses, instinct, and heart know that all too well. Have you ever seen a person that intuitively wants to lead themselves into terrible decisions?

What other people say about your intuition is irrelevant to how effective it is. You're the only person you have to convince. If you can't even do that at, then your gift becomes a curse, right down to its core.

To gain more confidence in your gut feeling, some retrospection is required. Look back at some good life decisions you've made. Don't forget to be thankful for what those decisions have brought you. Using your vivid imagination and memory, try to remember what you were feeling when you made those decisions.

What was your instinct telling you? Go back to that time and verify if your intuition served you well. Most likely, you will find that your gut was telling you it was good as well. You'll be surprised to know how accurate your instinct can be.

You may also be wondering about bad decisions in your life. Did you also follow your intuition during those times? Did you gut and instinct lead you astray? You may be inclined to blame your intuition for getting you into trouble as well, but that's only because you're missing on things.

During the times that you made poor decisions, were you only relying on your intuition? Take a closer look. Did you also let the opinions of other people affect your judgment? Were there other factors involved?

How about your other feelings? Were you hungry, sad or desperate when you made these decisions?

Sometimes, because of doubt, we try to find logical reasons to support our intuitions. This may or may not be the best idea. Finding a logical reason to back up a decision your instinct tells you to be right may not be the best idea at times.

Don't try to back up your gut feeling with more reasons. There will be times that those two won't mix and you'll end up twice as confused. This will dilute your resolution and lead you to half-baked solutions that won't do you any good.

10 - Understanding The Confusion

Where do you draw the line between intuitive thinking and hoping for the best? Fortunately, these two things share one core focus; the outcome.

How do you view the outcome of a certain situation? Here is where you get to test your intuition. Do you feel something will happen? Or do you want something to happen?

Sometimes, you could be blinded by your needs that we misunderstand what your intuition is telling you. You could really be hurting for the money, which is why you might tend to think that a shady business deal looks like a lifesaver. You could be lonely and depressed, which could lead you to think a friendship with a certain character could be beneficial for you.

When this happens, we tend to ignore what our gut is telling us. In turn, we mistake these needs as our intuition speaking to us, telling us to preserve ourselves and jump into something that may not be good for us.

When things go sour, we end up blaming our "poor" instincts and wish we knew better. If this has ever happened to you, it has to change now lest you repeat those mistakes despite having earnest and pure intentions.

Harboring A Desire

This central notion is what separates intuition and wishful thinking. Although desiring something in life is an inherently good thing, channeling all our focus and determination on this specific desire may not help us achieve this outcome.

Take, for instance, a cheating ex for whom you still have affection. Should this person ask for another shot at a relationship with you, what will your intuition say?

Naturally, the history of cheating will be a prevalent factor. There is proof of infidelity. This will certainly cause your intuition to tell you that getting back together is a bad idea.

However, your affection and desire to be happy with this person interfere with your better judgment. Although this is a classic contrast between the mind and the heart, the presence of a harbored desire makes things more complicated.

It's not conceited if you're wondering. Humans are just built that way. A life without a longing for something is not a life lived at all. What's important is that we use this desire to create purpose in our lives, and not let our yearnings cloud our judgment.

Separating Knowing From Wanting

It's unwise to purge yourself of desires that could cloud your judgment. Even the most dedicated monks need further clarity in their beliefs. You would be a completely different person without desires of any nature.

This is where your true empathic nature will arise. Being able to tell apart your desires and your hunches are the mark of a true intuitive. To do that, you need the firm habit of retrospection.

This is simply the habit of taking a step back and examining yourself through an emotional perspective. Here, you ask yourself a series of questions that will help you unearth the true nature of your feelings.

- Do I feel good about this because I want it?

- Am I jumping into this too quickly?

You can ask yourself any question to get to the heart of the issue. What's important is that you're aware of what you want and what your body is telling you. It's good if they're the same thing but never overlook the possibility that they might be very different.

As an intuitive, you probably already have this habit. The trick here is to place a goal at the start of your retrospection. Don't just verify what you're feeling. Try to segregate your desires from your intuition so that you can commit to something with all your heart.

The Fear of Vulnerability

On a fundamental level, your intuition serves a specific purpose; to save yourself. Along with the many other abilities that come with this talent, your instinct is designed to deter you from harming yourself.

On that same level, it can be said that it follows the natural state of humans to avoid pain. It's part of what makes us human. It's what makes us mortal. We value this mortality and ensure that we don't shorten our existence by our own accord.

As an intuitively gifted individual, this desire to stay safe becomes magnified, just like any other feeling you possess. You feel it a little more than everyone else. This also means you cherish it on a higher level as well.

With that said, your appreciation of a safe and comfortable environment immediately shows in your mood. At the same time, when something threatens your safety and well-being, you're one of the first people to show that fear.

It is that vulnerability that can hinder you from reaching your full potential as an intuitive. This is one of the first things you have to overcome in order to hone your instinct.

Accepting Vulnerability

What pushes us away from our weaknesses the most is the prospect of them damaging us in ways we clearly imagine. On that note, an intuitive does more than just imagine their vulnerabilities getting the best of them. They feel what it's like; and its unbearable for them.

Because of their sensitivities, intuitive people are more prone to shying away from exposing their weaknesses. They guard it with their very lives, only permitting a select few to get to know them well.

With all that being said, you'll be surprised to know that you can still find strength in being vulnerable. It just takes a different perspective.

According to psychology experts, we humans are predisposed to hate showing weakness. It's just not in our nature.

It makes us seem untrustworthy and unlovable. These are the last two things anyone would want for themselves.

But then again, what do you have to lose when you let other people know that you need them? What exactly happens to someone when they reveal their vulnerabilities? What comes after the terrifying thought of someone letting you down and leaving you to your fears?

This is what most people fail to see. We can be so shrouded in our fears that we no longer see what we stand to gain when we let other people in and show them that we need them.

We win lasting relationships. We win the kind of people we want in our lives; people that understand and accept us and our gifts. We get people who are just as willing to adjust to our needs as we are capable to adjust to theirs.

On that same note, we also filter out the people we don't need. We get to see who can be there for us and who can't. What's after that is a strong network you trust. What you get is a circle of meaningful relationships that will help you grow as a person. That is worth the fear.

No, that won't be easy by any means. After all, you have to

break a few eggs to make an omelet. Yes, it will hurt. Yes, you will be let down. Not everyone you let in will be worth the trouble, but that's where your intuition comes in.

Be careful of the people you let in, but don't shut everyone out for fear of getting hurt. It's alright to be scared, but it's never fine to live in constant fear. Yes, our fear is natural and born from our struggles and past failures. But with that said, it is our lasting relationships and bonds that make us human.

How To Overcome Fear

It's not enough just to be careful. Do you even have the strength and will to start? One thing about highly intuitive people is that they set up a barrier around themselves that no one else sees.

When you live in that barrier long enough, you tend to forget how to take it down when the right people come around. You become so enveloped in lonely comfort that you would rather live with what you have than enrich your life in the company of other people. That's one thing that makes it difficult to understand you.

To your surprise, it doesn't take an extraordinary individual to break down those walls. As much as you're yearning for relationships that breach your barriers, it is you that has to take them down. That is easier said than done.

The first thing you need to do is to stop overthinking.

Highly intuitive people can be very imaginative. For them, a simple meeting isn't just a pleasant experience. It's a sign of many great adventures with someone. It's a collection of happy memories waiting to be made.

You're not melodramatic, though. You just like thinking ahead to all the good times you'll be having with someone. That doesn't just apply to romantic relationships. You do the same thing with potential friendships.

When you start peering into the future, you start creating these mental images of what you want to happen with your bonds and where you want to take them. You suddenly make plans in your head and jump into conclusions.

Stop for a while and have yourself a reality check. Here, mindfulness meditation works wonders. When you start getting carried away by your instinct and imagination, take a breather and root yourself in the moment.

When you fail to stop yourself from thinking too far ahead, you end up making unrealistic expectations for these people which is a sure-fire way to become disappointed and miserable.

No, you're not controlling and manipulative. You're just hopeful and positive. That can be a good thing but only up to a certain extent. Keep your feet rooted and simply enjoy what you have at the moment. There will be a time for you to think of future adventures.

The next thing you need to learn is empathy.

Yes, you have needs in a relationship and bond with someone. Sure, you have requirements that certain people seem to meet at the moment. Despite that, you're not the only one who could badly need a meaningful connection.

Before you find the courage to let someone in, you need to learn what it means to be let in as well. Don't be clouded by your own needs that you fail to see how your presence is important to other people as well.

Don't forget that your needs come with a set of talents and sensitivities that make you a great companion and friend for other people. Use your gifts to create meaningful relationships with other people that need it.

When you experience what it's like being there for someone, you'll better appreciate what it's like when someone is there for you. You'll value this bravery more than ever, making you look over your fear of being vulnerable.

The last thing you have to learn is to communicate your need.

It doesn't come as simply saying "I need you in my life."

It usually doesn't even have to be a short and powerful statement that grabs the spotlight. Asking someone to be there for you doesn't have to be such a dramatic event. You can get your message across to the right people with a series of meaningful statements that hit the right spots.

- "Thank you for the time. I really needed that talk."

- "Thanks for seeing me today. I could really use a friend."

- "Your encouragement really helped me today."

- "I am very entertained by our discussions."

- "I look forward to our meetings and exchanges every

time."

As you can see from these statements, one sentiment stands out the most; gratitude.

Be thankful for the people that enrich your life. They are there for a reason. One thing people are so good at doing is overlooking the small things and over-dramatizing the big things.

Very few people understand the power of gratitude. When we are thankful for something, we rid ourselves of any fear or negative intention within ourselves. It's like cleaning our slates and realigning our focus towards more positive ventures.

When we are thankful, we attract better things towards ourselves. When other people see that, they become more comfortable around us and in turn, become part of our lives.

Being thankful is one way to attract the right people into your life. Never think about what one relationship means for you. Instead, think of what your relationship with this person could mean for them.

You may be intuitive, but you'll never know what it's like to be someone else once you've walked in their shoes. You may gain glimpses of their personal struggles and affairs, but the only way you'll get more depth is when someone lets you in.

You don't have to be direct with what you need. Simply be thankful and others will see that you cherish whatever bond you have with them. Once you've done that, you're bringing yourself closer to the right people without even realizing it. Sooner or later, your fear of becoming vulnerable with someone fades away and drowns in a sea of trust and positivity.

11 - A Life of Compassion and Wanting the Best

One very big part of being intuitive is the need to make the right decisions. The word "right" itself has a very deep meaning for you. It's the first thing you yearn when you get your inklings.

Because of the way you handle your emotions, it's natural for you to want what's best for everyone concerned. It's not a matter of principle. It's a matter of your talents.

Because you can sense what others could be feeling at a given moment, you take it upon yourself to make sure everyone is happy. This natural compassion may take you to great heights, and may also cause you great frustration.

Wanting What's Right

Despite your ability to notice if something's wrong, you can easily get stuck pondering on what would be beneficial for everyone. An interesting facet of an intuitive individual is that they are inherently compassionate and sharp at the same time.

You're well-designed to detect deception but your heart is

that of a humanitarian. This interesting contrast makes up most of your life struggles as an intuitive.

Finding the right mix between righteous and merciful can be a daunting task for the gifted intuitive. Sometimes, it even gets to the point wherein you take on the problems of other people as your own because you can feel their pain on a certain level.

This is where you have to learn how to pick your battles. It starts with accepting a single notion:

Your happiness and contentment will not come from solving everyone's problems. At times, what is best for everyone may not include your needs. So you end up sacrificing on your end just to please everyone but you end up with the short end of the stick. This leaves you defeated.

But you can't help it. You know the satisfaction of doing the right thing more than anyone else because of your gift.

You can't please everyone, even if you think you're doing what's right for everyone. Sure, your intuition tells you what is right, but that may not be the same idea shared by the people you're trying to help.

You have a deeper understanding compared to other people. It's best not to expect people to see things the way you do. The sooner you realize and accept this universal truth, the lighter you'll feel when you walk away from events that are out of your control. Sometimes, the right thing to do is to mind your own business.

But you have to want it to make it worthwhile. As an intuitive individual, you detest the notion of giving up on something, especially when you've dedicated yourself. You have to draw the line between doing what's right for everyone and preserving your own happiness. You're special, alright; but you're not a superhero.

It is when you see the emotional plight of other people that you forget to treasure your own balance. When that happens, you dive deep into someone else's affairs with the intent of helping them.

Before doing that, take a step back and do some retrospection and self-assessment. Learn to love yourself a little when you feel the need to take on someone else's problems.

12 - Understanding Bodily Cues

In line with living with your gift, it's important to be attuned to the way your body operates. Regardless of the type of intuition you receive, it is important to recognize the signs your body gives you when it is trying to tell you something.

Even if your intuition works by giving you images, your body will still try to give you hints about a certain situation. Take note that your intuition is not rooted in your conscious mind. It dances in your subconscious. It happens even if you don't tell your body; just like breathing.

On that same train of thought, take a good look at yourself in certain situations. You can also go back to specific events in your life and review the way you behaved and how your body interacted with you.

Do you notice certain habits that come out of you in certain situations? What were the nature of those events? What sensations flooded you during those times? As you answer these questions, write them down in your journal to keep track of your progress.

Positive Signs

Start with the good events in your life. They don't have to be big, important undertakings such as weddings and work promotions. Your intuitive body also sends signals during the simplest joys in life; such as a short afternoon chat with a friend over coffee.

Although different intuitive individuals have different ways their bodies communicate with them, experts point out to a few commonalities that stand out during positive events.

Primarily, your shoulders tend to relax during good times as an indicator that everything is going smoothly. They aren't tensed and raised in anticipation of a threat.

If you're with someone with whom you're comfortable, you also tend to lean towards their direction. When you're enjoying a good conversation, which seems to be going in interesting directions, your body shows its interest as well by optimizing your position to hear well and understand more efficiently.

Another thing to note is that your breathing tempo is normalized. You're not hyperventilating from stress because your body isn't intercepting any potential threat to you.

You will note that breathing can be either a conscious or unconscious effort. When your body delegates breathing to your subconscious, it becomes a great indicator of your current state.

Finally, one of the biggest signs of positive times ahead is the presence of goosebumps. This happens when you're anxious about something good or influential. You may have experienced these at the onset of something really good or right in the middle of something nice as it happens.

When your body intuitively does these things, it's time to relax further in the knowledge that everything is going to be alright.

Negative Signs

If your body communicates to you in the presence of good times, then it also has warning signs that tell you something is amiss. Experts have also found some common behaviors our bodies use to tell us to double back and reexamine our situations.

First, if breathing is normalized during good times because of your subconscious comfort, it then becomes restricted and hampered when your body is perceiving a threat to your well-being.

Interestingly, you hold your breath unknowingly at certain points as if to brace yourself for something shocking or unwelcome. This can also be accompanied by a tightening of the throat which makes breathing a more difficult task.

Another sign is the iconic chill down the spine. It may or may not be a cold wind going down your back, but your spine shivers from a rush of hormones coming from your central nervous system.

On top of that, you can also feel discomfort in your stomach. These aren't the butterflies you expect during romantic affairs, but a sinking and twisting feeling urging you to go to the bathroom and reexamine yourself.

Along with those, your body could also alert you to old wounds and other ailments you may have. You could have a sudden headache or an old scab would start twitching.

When your body uses pain to get your attention, it's usually because you're subconsciously anticipating a worst-case scenario and your action is required immediately.

These are just a few ways your body speaks to you. The more you listen, the better message you'll get from your intuition. Hence, it is important to keep a journal so that you can log your various states throughout the day. This is the only way you can effectively learn how your body tells you things.

Stress For The Highly Intuitive

Besides signals, your body also responds to stress differently from other people. What may stress others may not be so bothersome to you. On that same note, what could be dauntingly stressful for you may not seem like a big issue for other people.

This is why you should be aware of what triggers your stress reactions. For a gifted intuitive such as yourself, you're probably to incur stress from a certain number of things.

One of the foremost triggers of your stress is the need to do what's right all the time. This may be an easy choice at times, but when it requires a little more digging and some trial and error, it becomes frustrating.

This is especially true when you have multiple decisions to make at the same time. This could happen when you're planning a vacation with your friends or deciding what movie to see with some of your relatives.

In another sense, you're also a perfectionist. Because of your sensitivity to yourself, you know what it feels when you don't give 100% of yourself to a certain task. When you can't consider your work to be perfect, it gets to you. You then question your capabilities regardless of what other people are saying.

Another thing that triggers your stress reactions is your propensity to overthink.

Being highly intuitive, you can't help but learn new things about yourself. You give great priority to experiences that teach you knew things about yourself and the people around you.

In turn, you begin to worry about almost everything you do, no matter how mundane the task is. This is because the mind of an intuitive individual is a very active one. It may be full of impulsive thoughts and sentiments, but that doesn't mean it's not at work. You just don't see the ticking clocks and gears inside your head but they're there, spinning around like there's no tomorrow.

And this could cause a lot of worry for you. Combined with your tendency to be perfect, you could end up constantly questioning the purpose of the things you do and the manner in which you're doing them.

This puts you in a state of constant self-checking. Without proper de-stressing methods, you could end up suffering from chronic stress even without the interference of other people.

To counteract this, experts suggest the implementation of meaningful rituals throughout the day to help you appease the internal cynic within.

One of these rituals is to meditate in the morning. It doesn't have to a religious experience. It just has to be a unifying one that sets all your worries aside and shifts your energy from tense to relaxed.

Try setting aside at least fifteen minutes in the morning to meditate and clear your thoughts. One of the best things you can do at this time is some mindfulness meditation.

This is especially helpful when your day doesn't start out the way you wanted. When you wake up to demands and complaints and other concerns, you know things are going to get rough.

They get rougher when your mind and body aren't prepared to meet the challenges of the day. This short morning ritual will help you get your head in the game and help you maintain your focus.

Eating Right

It's only natural that the food you eat also affects the way your body communicates with you. Your food choices shouldn't just revolve around the notion of being physically fit. Your diet has to also help keep your intuition sharp.

After years of study, psychics and healing gurus have determined that your intuition and instinct rely on your endocrine glands to alert your body and keep your senses sharp. This is why you should make it a point to ingest food items that will promote the growth and proper maintenance of these glands.

For that, your first choice should be pineapples. It's important not to go for the canned variety which could contain unhealthy preservatives. You will want the fresh kind of pineapple.

Be careful not to just rely on pineapple juice, though. Consuming the fruit isn't just a sweet and refreshing treat. It also enriches your endocrine glands. Many experts believe that pineapples are also a source of psychic energy, helping you clear your mind as you tap into your intuition.

Another suitable choice is broccoli. Scientists have found that organic broccoli helps stimulate the operation of your endocrine glands. When these are healthy, your body becomes better at releasing hormones into your bloodstream, immediately alerting you of your intuitions.

On a more nutritional level, you will also want to get a good dose of vitamins A and D at the same time. These nutrients are known to interact well with your endocrine system, allowing for a better synthesis of your hormones.

In that sense, almond nuts and Brazil nuts are ideal sources of this combination. Couple those with daily intakes of dairy products such as milk and cheese, and you have a healthy set of endocrine glands.

13 - The Intuitive Dreamer

Most people simply dismiss dreams and patched-up scraps of memories that seem to bind themselves together when you sleep. For the intuitive individual though, dreams play a very significant role when it comes to understanding their emotions.

This is probably the reason why intuitive people enjoy vivid dreams more often than most people. When you dream of something good, you sense every details and take away the joy long after you wake up.

The same thing can be said about nightmares. They glare into your being and haunt you with their mysterious meanings even when you're no longer sleeping. This is why gifted intuitive people pay very close attention to their dreams. Once you learn how to read your dreams, their messages will empower you and help you live your gifted life to the fullest.

Dream Interpretation

Fortunately, you don't need a third eye or years of experience as an empath or psychic to understand what your dreams mean for you. All you need is some basic knowledge and some simple recording tools.

With that said, the most important thing you'll need is your journal. How can you analyze a dream if you don't write it down? Sadly, humans are prone to forgetting most of their dreams a few minutes after they wake up. Intuitive people, however, can maintain these memories after they're awake, allowing them to better recall them when the time comes.

Keep your journal beside you when you go to sleep. When you wake up from a dream, reach for the journal and scribble down what happened in your dream.

Don't try to immediately dissect your dream as you write. The goal is to get as much of what you've dreamed onto paper for later inspection. Do not worry about being chronologically correct of the events that take place in your dreams. You will want to get as many details as possible.

What To Ask Yourself

After a dream as well as your efforts to write them in your journal, find time within the day to sit down with your work. There, go over the things that transpired in your mind and try to see if you can play things back based on your notes.

As you go over these notes, ask yourself some questions which will help you discern what your subconscious is trying to tell you.

What was the theme?

Look back at your memory of the dream and try to see if there was a general theme for what happened. Here, you try to determine if you had a good dream or bad dream.

Each event that took place in your dream revolves around a certain effect. Despite being unorganized and chaotic, our subconscious still manages to organize our dreams around a central concept. Were you dreaming of a celebration? A test? An attack? A death? A romance? Zero in on that concept.

To help you answer that question, try to take apart various elements of your dream and ask yourself more specific questions. Where were you in the dream? Are you familiar with the place? Who was with you? What were you doing with these people? Was there anything happening to you?

Were you reliving a good memory? Or a bad one? Try to factor our details that are too hazy for you to remember and focus on the things that came vividly. Did any particular object or person stand out from the things that happened in your dream?

As you answer this question, write your sentiments down as well. Those will soon come together in the form of a message as you complete your dream analysis.

What was the predominant emotion?

What was the general mood of the events that took place in your dream? Don't just try to remember what mood the people and atmosphere had. Look back and try to determine what emotions you yourself were feeling in your dream?

Don't just say happy if you were happy. Here is where things get interesting. Try to rationalize the way you were feeling in your dream. If you felt happy during the dream, try to tell yourself why you were feeling that way.

Was it because you were with someone? Was it because something favorable to you was happening in your dream? Was it because of the other people involved in the dream? Did you win something? Did you get rid of something? Try to a "why" to what you were feeling.

Even if you were feeling something negative, it's still important to rationalize. If you were feeling terrified by your dream, try to zero in on what triggered your fear. Were you being attacked? Was someone close to you being attacked? Was something important to you being destroyed? Were you the one being destroyed? Was something being taken from you?

Answering these questions will help you understand a little more about yourself. Perhaps there is something that you can't admit to yourself when you're awake which causes your subconscious to reflect your true sentiments while you sleep.

What symbols were present in the dream?

Don't just look for insignia, flags, and signs in your dream. The word "symbol" can be a very vague term at times.

When looking for symbols, look for things, actions, gestures and even people that stuck out to you. An important symbol in your dream is one that usually stands out the most and is what you can immediately recall when you wake up.

Were you at the amusement park? Did you ride nothing but

the roller coaster? Were you celebrating someone's birthday or wedding? Did you give them something? Was something given to you?

Were you with someone in your dream? What were you doing with this person? What was this person doing to you? What does this person mean to you?

Sadly, there are no defined sets of characteristics to tell you what makes a symbol in your dream. It's more of a personal question. What was symbolic to you? What element of your dream do you believe signifies something that translates into your waking world?

When you've found your symbols, be sure to write them down and highlight their seeming importance to you. Don't worry if you can't put a finger on their significance yet, the activity isn't over.

How are all these elements connected?

When you have the theme, symbols, and emotions written down, you're ready to start digging deep.

Put on your thinking cap and awaken the left side of your brain. Here, you're also going to need logic to put everything together in a central message. Take the various elements you've dissected and try to piece them together into one central message. What are these things, feelings, people and emotions trying to tell me?

Take, for example, a dream about you standing in front of a classroom, without any clothes on.

The first and most striking emotion you'll experience is a shame. The embarrassment will almost overwhelm you. This shame is symbolic for you because it stands out the most.

Take this as a sign that you might be walking into an embarrassing situation. It could be at work or with your friends and family. Whatever it is, the shame will almost be unbearable.

Take it as your brain trying to tell you what you're going to feel if you don't take action. Try to remember the people laughing and you and pointing at you as you stand in front of them naked. It's all one big symbol revolving around the concept of shame that puts you in the spotlight.

Take note that this is not the only rationale behind interpreting dreams. It happens to be a very personal experience. It requires a delicate combination of tracing back your past experiences and the sensations you feel as you dream.

Only you can tell the significance of the symbols you encounter in the dream world. This is why it's important to let your thoughts fly as you ponder on the supposed meaning of these symbols to you.

It's important not to force a connection. Just let your thoughts and imagination run lose as you think about it. Make sure your mind is relaxed. It's a good idea to practice some mindfulness meditation right before engaging in this activity.

This is where the final step and question comes in. What actionable course can I take?

Once you have the message, what are you going to do about it? Once you have the interpretation, it's time to put things into action. It's time to take the subconscious message and place it in your conscious plans.

Going back to your humiliating example, you can start by either reviewing any work you might have submitted or will yet be submitted. Double check if you've made any grave errors that could cost you your competence.

Don't just take a look at your work. Go back on your social media newsfeeds and post and see if you haven't been making a fool of yourself in front of other people on the internet.

14 - Conclusion

As you complete this manual, notice that you've become more comfortable with yourself and your talents. Congratulations on reaching a new level of appreciating your gift!

The first thing you will want to do after this is to get your journal. If you have one already prior to this manual, go ahead and write about your experience reading this book. What points struck close to home? What new concepts were introduced? What new discoveries did you make about yourself?

If you're only starting a journal after this book, make your first entry a special one by committing to writing in it every day.

Don't just set aside a certain time of day in which to write. Commit to writing what goes on in your heart and in your mind the moment something interesting happens to you. Write in it the moment you are plagued by your emotions and instinct.

What's important here is that you begin to like writing in your journal. It won't solidify as a habit if you don't appreciate what it does for you.

For your first entry, write about how you feel, now that you've uncovered much of this great talent that lies deep inside you. Does it empower you to become more confident? Or does it confuse you to think that you still have much to learn? No matter what you're feeling, root yourself in the moment and register it to memory.

When you've done that, it's time to go out into the world and share your gifts with the people who matter most. You may have family members already going through something that needs your understanding and advice. You may have friends that need a listening ear. Go out and build those bonds to further empower your talents.

Also, don't forget that you're not the only gifted intuitive individual on the planet. Seek like-minded and like-gifted people. Meet them and learn from them. You will be amazed at how deep and complex other intuitive people can be from the eyes of another intuitive person.

On the same note, don't be afraid to share what you know about your gift to other individuals that are struggling with their intuition. Be a beacon for them and show them the path to truly enjoying the gift.

14 - CONCLUSION

Congratulations once again!

Thank You

As we reach the end of this book, I want to say thanks for reading this book.

I want to get this information out to as many people as possible. If you found this book helpful, I would greatly appreciate you leaving me a review. This helps others find the book as well.

Disclaimer

This document is geared towards providing exact and reliable information in regards to the topic and issue covered. The publication is sold on the idea that the publisher is not required to render an accounting, officially permitted, or otherwise, qualified services. If advice is necessary, legal, financial, medical or professional, a practiced individual in the profession should be ordered.

This information is not presented by a financial or medical practitioner and is for entertainment, educational and informational purposes only. The content is not intended as a substitute for professional medical advice, diagnosis, or treatment. Always seek the advice of your physician or other qualified health care provider with any questions you may have regarding a medical condition. Never disregard professional medical advice or delay in seeking it because of something you have read.

The information provided herein is stated to be truthful and consistent, in that any liability, in terms of inattention or otherwise, by any usage or abuse of any policies, processes, or directions contained within is the solitary and utter responsibility of the recipient reader. Under no circumstances will any legal responsibility or blame be held against the

DISCLAIMER

publisher for any reparation, damages, or monetary loss due to the information herein, either directly or indirectly.

Last Updated: 29.Sep.2017